What people are saying about

Our Bodies Stay Home, Our Imaginations Run Free

CONGRATULATIONS!! Your book is FANTASTIC! It brought me to tears. This fabulous new book is so valuable for children in numerous ways. It beautifully incorporates a full range of emotions, thoughts, experiences, worries and considerable concerns through a story of a close family as they follow Coronavirus stay-at-home recommendations. The story artfully reflects a child's need to grasp an understanding for new practices and family routines. The highlight of the book is the surprise that takes place at the end. This wonderful book brought welcomed heartwarming tears.

—-Deborah McNelis, M.Ed, Founder, Brain Insights, LLC

In a time when young children are confused and anxious about the sudden changes in their lives, Ms. Hyler has expertly found a way to explain the science of COVID-19 in a way that does not make children feel like victims, but instead empowers them to do their part to flatten the curve and slow the spread. Her upbeat story about a young girl having a birthday while social distancing is a necessity encourages a positive outlook about being creative and finding innovative and fun ways to embrace our new normal.

—Diane H. Munzenmaier, PhD, Program Director,
Professional Development in STEM Education,
Center for BioMolecular Modeling,
Milwaukee School of Engineering

Lora Hyler has written a story that embraces children, providing both comfort and instruction for families learning to navigate this new and uncertain time. Thank you Lora, for this book.

—Justen Ahren, Former Martha's Vineyard Poet Laureate,
Poet, Photographer, Musician, Writing Workshop Facilitator

This important new book is a well-written fictional interpretation of one family's effort to deal with the local and global impact of Covid-19. The detailed and diverse cover illustration is a powerful reminder that this virus IS global, even though the story is firmly anchored in an American urban setting.

The struggles of the Thomas family are presented as specific to their own situation but also common to a vast community. Despite the wider impact of a pandemic, young Maya and her brother Bryan experience typical sibling stresses and reactions with lively scenes and dialogue. That familiarity allows informative and supportive parental roles to play out naturally, including meltdowns, virtual school sessions, reminders, and applied advice about safe practices and routines. Within this simple story the focus is on responsible and creative ways to adjust, for small events and large (including a birthday!), to a new way of life within a familiar, loving, and secure setting. Daily roller-coaster emotions are credible and helpful for readers young and old.

The public health benefit of a short, direct story like this is immeasurable, and will prove welcome to families and educators.

—Sandy Brehl, Author, Society of Children's Book Writers and Illustrators –
Wisconsin Member, Retired Elementary Educator

Lora Hyler's latest novel is a beautiful depiction of the early days of the coronavirus pandemic, filled with joy for the things in life that really matter: the love of family and friends, the support of community and gratitude for good health. Through Maya Thomas, we witness everyone's anxiety about the disease and hope for the future.

—Jerod Santek, Artistic Director
Write On, Door County

Let your own imagination run free as you learn about how (almost-8-year old) Maya and her family handled their ups and downs during the Covid-19 pandemic. Get your questions answered about how you, too, can stay safe. Along the way, get inspired by creative ideas, ways to connect, and positivity. Lora Hyler's OUR BODIES STAY HOME, OUR IMAGINATIONS RUN FREE will provide ways to help you through challenges as you stay home to stay safe. Great story!

—Joyce Uglow, Webinar Coordinator
Society of Children's Book Writers and Illustrators – Wisconsin

Our Bodies Stay Home,
Our Imaginations Run Free

A Coronavirus Covid-19 Story for Children

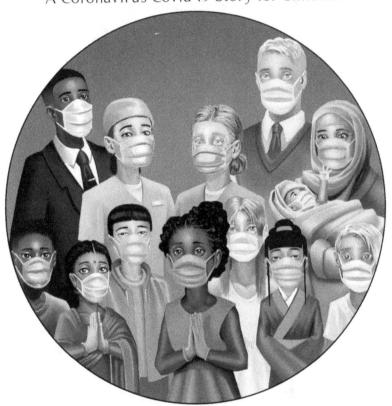

Lora L. Hyler

Also by Lora L. Hyler

The Stupendous Adventures of Mighty Marty Hayes

Our Bodies Stay Home, Our Imaginations Run Free

A Coronavirus Covid-19 Story for Children

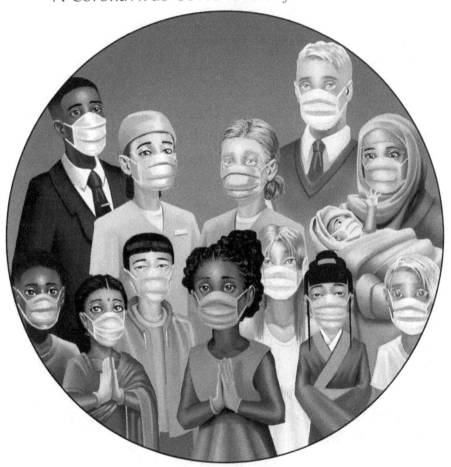

Lora L. Hyler

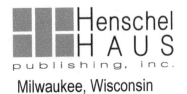

Henschel
HAUS
publishing, inc.
Milwaukee, Wisconsin

Published by
HenschelHAUS Publishing, Inc.
www.henschelHAUSbooks.com
Please contact the publisher for quantity
and non-profit discounts: info@henschelHAUSbooks.com

ISBN: 978159598-774-7
E-ISBN: 978159598-775-4
LCCN: 2020938696

Cover and interior art: Ian Wade, Instagram.com/dracanimaart

I dedicate this work to my family and extended family,
along with every reader braving the coronavirus.
Who writes a book during a pandemic?

My inspiration was an Emory Global Health Institute competition to
help children understand why their lives had so quickly changed.
CEO Pamela Redmon wrote to authors, "Congratulations to ALL on
writing your book in the very short amount of time, and we hope you
will share your work with others."

I accepted the challenge of writing this book in less than ten days,
knowing children in my community are facing the pandemic with a
sense of loss, but also humor and laughter. I hope this story comforts
and delights them as much as their resilience inspires me.

ACKNOWLEDGMENTS

Scientists, doctors and the entire medical community are working hard to keep us safe. We can't forget our spiritual leaders and wellness gurus who are assisting with our mental health in the face of a 100-year pandemic.

I'd like to acknowledge every person in my life who made it his or her mission to check in, contribute to community members needing help, and lean in with faith that "This too shall pass."

I know I'm not alone in learning to appreciate the soft hum of a world involuntarily locked in slow-down mode. It seems we received the gift of a "do over." With time to step away from our frantic world, we are learning to evaluate what's really important in our lives.

To the children who are showing us the way through their chalk messages of hope, window art, bubbling laughter, and bright-eyed smiles, I salute you.

I appreciate my husband of 29 years, Ken Pinckney, our son William, and our extended family and friends. Many are like family. You know who you are. Thank you to everyone who has accompanied me on this author journey.

Most of all, I thank my parents, Haward and Leona Hyler who, at a very early age, taught me the value of reading books.

Lora L. Hyler

May 2020

Maya Misses her Friends

Maya rolled over in bed. Her dancing clock was going off.

The face of the clock featured Kermit the frog, and the speaker belted out, "*It's not easy being green.*"

Who set the alarm? Big brother is back to his hijinks, Maya thought.

As she wiped the sleep from her eyes, she knew deep down something was different.

It wasn't a school day.

She wouldn't see her lunch lady.

She wouldn't get to bring her favorite art creation for Show-and-Tell.

And worst of all, she would miss seeing all her friends and her favorite teacher. She wanted to get back to second grade.

As her eyes brimmed with tears, she shook her head of braids and said aloud, "I may not see Mrs. Jackson in person, but we can talk on video chat."

"Maya, is that you?" A voice called from just outside her door.

"Yes, Bryan set my alarm again. It's not funny!" she screamed.

Maya's mom yelled behind her as she turned to go find her oldest child. "That boy, he needs to stop these pranks!"

Maya sighed as she rolled over. It was day 45 at home, and she wasn't sure what she was going to do to fill her day.

Then her mood brightened. It was Friday. The day Mrs. Jackson checked in on her.

The sound of clanging metal alerted Maya that she was about to be disturbed even more.

At the slightest sound, the family's goldendoodle would tear through the house and joyfully leap into the air to join her in bed.

She took a deep breath and braced for the happiest dog she knew. Harlan had heard her alarm and came running. Soon he launched himself into her bed, licking her face as if he hadn't seen her in weeks.

Maya giggled aloud, accepted his sloppy kisses, and caught a whiff of his breath. She grabbed her nose, "Harlan, what have you been eating? Is someone feeding you sausage again?"

She giggled again. Her mother always reminded her to think of all the happy things whenever she felt sad about how coronavirus had changed their lives.

"Harlan, Harlan, I'm just waking up," Maya protested. "OK, OK. I'm up. We might as well go downstairs and see what dad is up to."

Harlan took a running leap and jumped to the floor, speeding ahead of her to get downstairs for what he hoped were more treats.

Maya shook her head at her oversized dog. He thought he was still a puppy, but he weighed more than she did. She pulled on her robe and slippers and headed downstairs.

MAYA'S MELTDOWN

Maya's dad was already at his favorite spot in the kitchen, in front of the coffee maker. Maya could smell the nutty flavor of his favorite hazelnut coffee beans.

She smiled and grabbed a seat at the kitchen table. Bright sunlight flooded the room.

"Looks like it's going to be another beautiful day," Dad said.

"Yeah, I guess," Maya responded with a sigh.

Bryan entered the kitchen rapping, "Get back. Don't get all up on me…"

Their dad took a sip and raised an eyebrow. "I see Harlan could not wait to get you out of bed. And you, young man, must be working on your rap game again."

"It was Bryan!" Maya yelled, surprising herself. "He's always messing with me. I could have slept in."

"What are you talking about? We have lessons in a half hour," Bryan said.

As their mom rounded the corner into the kitchen, Maya burst into tears.

"Why can't things be like they were before the coronavirus? No school. No play dates. No building Legos with friends. No pizza parties or bowling. No visiting grandma and grandpa at their house. Everything is different!"

Mom and Dad exchanged looks. All that Maya said was true.

Maya's dad set down his coffee, walked over and put his arms around her. "I know this gets upsetting sometimes. I know you miss a lot of things. We all do. It's OK to be upset sometime."

"Just not all the time," Bryan countered.

"Bryan, now's not the time," Mom said. "Maya, do you want to talk about it?"

Maya sniffled. Harlan sat at her feet, and cocked his head, looking for a treat. "I just want to get back to my stuff." She held out her hands. "Even my hands are having a hard time."

Maya's dad walked back to get her a plate of food. He knew that homemade biscuits and gravy with a side of chicken sausage were her favorite.

Maya's mom grabbed her hands, and kissed her daughter on the forehead. "I have a cure for that. I'll share my special shea butter. I can't cure the coronavirus, sweetheart. But we can do our part. Washing our hands regularly for twenty seconds will help."

"Twenty seconds," Bryan said at the same time. "And I'm sorry for playing that alarm clock prank."

"The better we are at following the guidelines set by the doctors, the sooner we can get this coronavirus under control," Dad said, setting a plate in front of Maya. "This will end."

"Are you sure?" Maya asked as her tears continued to fall.

"I'm certain. Many of our best medical and scientific minds are working on this virus. It needs to pass from person to person to live, so the more we stay put and prevent it from entering our bodies, the quicker it will leave," he said.

"Dad, I get the handwashing part. Of course, if you touch something that the virus is sitting on, your hands are then infected. You could touch your face and have it enter your body that way," Bryan noted. "The part I don't get is the 'stay six feet away from other people' part."

"Mrs. Jackson said that's because somebody could sneeze on you or spit when they talk, and boom boom pow, you've got corona, just like that," Maya said, throwing up her hands.

"Coronavirus," Bryan said.

"This virus is part of a family of viruses called coronavirus. Covid-19 is the disease that results from it," Dad explained. "C-O for 'Corona, 'V-I for Virus and 19 for the year 2019, when it was first discovered."

"How did this start?" Maya asked.

"The scientists and doctors are still working to figure that out. They'll get better at dealing with it. We will learn how to best deal with this covid-19," Dad said.

"So, when are we going to get back to normal?" Maya asked, reaching for her food.

"One minute, young lady. Do you mind taking a quick trip to the bathroom and washing your hands before breakfast?"

Maya skipped off. Her dad slid the plate away from the edge of the table where it was tempting Harlan. The dog whimpered when he saw the plate moving away from him.

"I appreciate the extra chores you're taking on, son," Dad said, turning his attention to Bryan.

Bryan shrugged.

"No, I mean it. Every little bit helps. Washing your hands after playing with Harlan, before meals, after time outside, taking care to wash surfaces you come into contact with, wearing your mask in public. This all helps flatten the curve."

"I think I know what that means." Bryan sat down at the table and rolled up his sleeves.

"So, the cases of people infected with covid-19 peaks at some point in a community. We want the number of infections to flatten out and fall. We need to take care of infected folks and save these people," he added.

"Good job," mom said. "It took me a while to understand what Dr. Fauci was explaining in the national news conferences. You explained it better than I can."

Bryan beamed.

As Maya took her place back at the table, Harlan the goldendoodle cocked his head to one side and looked at her expectantly.

"What did I miss?" Maya asked.

"Did you remember to sing the *Happy Birthday* song twice, Maya?" Dad asked.

"Three times!" Maya said, taking a large bite of her gravy-drenched biscuit. "The more I wash, the quicker coronavirus leaves my town!"

The family laughed. Harlan joined in with a chorus of loud barking.

THE THOMAS FAMILY GOES FOR A WALK

It had taken some convincing, but the Thomas family had gotten in the habit of taking daily walks together. They usually went after 4 or 5 p.m. when Mom and Dad were finished with work and done helping Maya and Bryan with homework.

It was a great way for everyone to talk about their day, or just relax. They would spot life moving around in their wooded subdivision, both two-legged and four-legged creatures.

During the day, Bryan was perfectly comfortable spending time roaming between his room, and enjoying the lower level filled with exercise equipment. He also spent time on video calls with his friends and completing homework.

Maya had her homework and her chats with her favorite teacher, Mrs. Jackson. She lived for those days!

"We have to work to build up our immune systems," Mom would remind Bryan when he tried to get out of going on the walks. He thought the whole family walking together looked dorky.

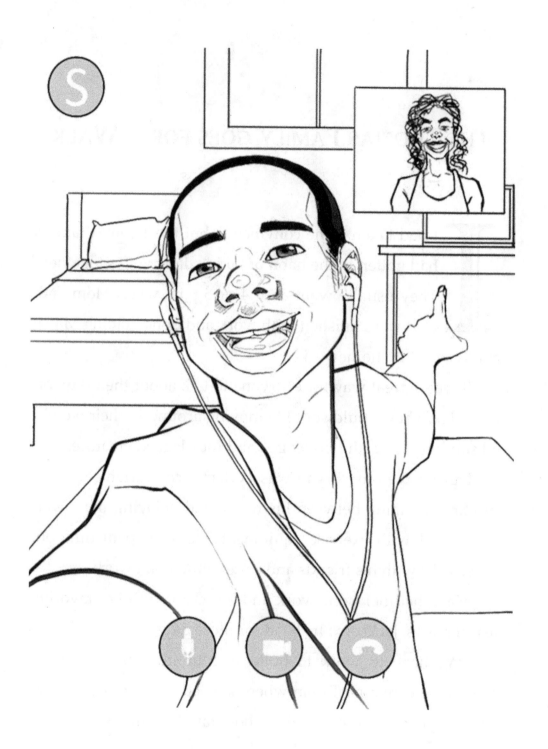

Maya was always eager to go. Each walk felt like an adventure! Who knew what they would spot in the wild?

On these walks, she noticed their busy subdivision was quieter than usual. Sure, there were the usual squeals of kids playing, but playtimes were in the kids' own yards and with their own family members.

No playmates. *Thanks, corona,* Maya thought to herself.

It seemed that during this time, her ears heard a lot better. Planes flying overhead were rare, and car traffic was down.

She could tell when the mail truck rounded the corner and headed toward their street. She knew the heavy sound of the garbage truck, the recycling truck, and the neighbor's motorcycle.

She spotted different kinds of birds on full display as they competed for seeds at her Dad's beloved bird feeders scattered around their backyard. Sparrows. Robins. Cardinals.

Walking around, she noticed neighbors had bird feeders, too.

Maya saw budded trees. Baby rabbits darted here and there. Wild turkeys roamed. The family would take care to steer clear. Turkeys are known to get cranky and follow folks walking. Some even chase folks on bicycles!

Chipmunks darted. Squirrels performed acrobatic tricks as they swung from tree to tree to get to their destination.

The family's walk route changed to refresh the time out together. Luckily there was a river just a few blocks away.

This gave them a beautiful park to explore, complete with a waterfall and benches for viewing. If they picked the right day, fishermen stood in waders casting their rods, hoping for the night's catch.

For Maya, the best part of the walk was spotting all the encouraging signs in windows of homes and seeing the new chalk art decorating driveways.

Sometimes balloons floated in the breeze, attached to mailboxes.

These happy signs were like a breath of fresh air. She wondered about the kids or adults who created the art.

Her favorites included:

Stay strong.

We are one.

It's OK to slow down and breathe.

Do like cats and dogs. Follow the joy.

Be kind.

Kindness always wins.

In a rut? Help somebody.

Pick some flowers and share love.

Call a friend if you're feeling down.

When in doubt, look for the helpers.

Some of the chalk art lasted for days, if there wasn't any rain. Others were there one day, gone the next.

Maya's mom smiled and nudged her until Maya's face blossomed into a toothy grin.

Maya thought to herself, *These walks are alright.*

Even Bryan had a skip in his step.

* * * * **

When the Thomas family returned home, Mom set up the computer.

"It's almost time for your grandparents to call us," she announced. The family gathered around the dining room table for their multi-generational video call. The kids were always excited to talk to their grandparents.

The screen lit up.

"Here are my grandbabies," a voice said. "Hi, Maya. Hi, Bryan. Hello, Mary and Ken."

"Hi, Grandma!" Maya and Bryan said together.

"It's so nice to talk to you, Mom and Dad. How are you?" Maya's mom asked.

"Other than missing you guys, we're great. I felt a little sad about not seeing you, so I had to put on my music today. Listen," Grandma said.

Amazing Grace, how sweet the sound...

The kids listened intently as their mom and dad smiled, placing their arms around one another.

Grandpa softly sang along. As the song came to an end, Grandma's favorite verse began,

Through many dangers, toils and snares, we have already come,
'Twas Grace that brought us safe thus far,
And Grace will lead us home.

"My favorite song never fails me. Kids, I know the language may seem a bit ole-timey, but let me tell you what it means during this time. Amazing Grace lets us know this isn't the first trouble to come our way. Us older folks have been through a lot."

"You can say that again," Grandpa said.

"And we'll go through much more. Hopefully, not anything this upsetting in your lifetime. The lyricist who wrote *Amazing*

Grace set out to carry us through tough times and to remind us to be strong," Grandma said, pointing her finger at the screen.

"Did you hear Grace will lead us home? What that means to me is we have help getting through this. Don't despair. We will be alright."

"I love this song, and I love you, Grandma. I want to hug you soon," Maya said softly.

"We can't wait to hug you too, baby. We'll do our favorite activities and eat our favorite ice cream," Grandpa said with a smile.

"Cookie dough!" Maya shouted.

"Vanilla with sprinkles!" Bryan yelled.

"Hot fudge sundae for me," Dad said. "And a strawberry sundae for Mom."

"I have an idea!" Maya shouted. "For our next call, how about if we all get our favorite ice cream from the store and eat it during our call?"

"Works for me," Bryan said.

"Let's do it!" Grandpa said.

Everyone nodded with big smiles on their faces.

Harlan lay at Maya's feet. She could have sworn his ears perked up at the mention of ice cream.

Birthday Plans?

The next day, Maya's mom took a noon break from her work. She set her computer aside and went to find Maya and Bryan.

Bryan was in the middle of a video call with his best friend, Ted, so she searched for Maya.

Maya was curled up in her bed, a book on her lap.

"Maya, how about a round of ladder game outside before we get lunch?"

"What are we having?" Maya asked, peeping over her book.

"Homemade pizza. With whatever toppings you guys want. I cut them up and set them aside last night. The dough's ready, just make and bake."

"Cool. I want pepperoni and veggies."

"Done."

"Let's get some fresh air."

Maya set her book aside, and they strolled through their patio doors to the backyard with Harlan at their feet.

Harlan immediately stretched his legs and circled the yard, no doubt searching for squirrels to chase.

Mom handed out the bolas and the game began.

The ladder game is simple. Three rungs on a plastic ladder frame, three balls on a short rope (bolas). Three throws per player. And a simple scoring system.

Maya went first, throwing each of her three bolas. Her aim was off. One landed on the bottom rung for one point. The other two plopped straight to the ground.

Mom noticed Maya looked deep in thought. "Someone's a little preoccupied."

"I was just wondering what kind of birthday party I'll have next week," Maya said softly.

Her mom cleared her throat, tossed her braids, and took a deep breath. "A creative one."

Mom began to throw her three bolas. The first one landed on the top rung—three points. Second throw, also three points, and third throw, two points landing on the middle rung.

"A creative one," Maya repeated. "What does that mean, Mom?"

"It means we'll figure it out. We don't know what it will look like, but we will celebrate. We will celebrate your birth. We will celebrate our health. And we will include our family and friends as much as we're able."

"Video calls?" Maya asked.

"Technology is a beautiful thing, baby."

Our Bodies Stay Home, Our Imaginations Run Free

"I was thinking, Mom, maybe this birthday shouldn't be about me. I know kids are helping fight coronavirus. They're making masks, running errands for old folks in the neighborhood, and calling friends and family to make sure they're OK."

Maya's mom was surprised to hear Maya sound so wise. She ran her hand through her braids. "That's true."

"Maybe we can do something," Maya suggested. "We see a lot of people on our walks and walking their dogs past our house. We could have a sale and raise money to buy masks, or make the masks ourselves."

"We'll figure it out."

Maya smiled. This too shall pass, her mom always said. They just needed to find a good way to help their community. *Our bodies stay home. Our imaginations run free.*

Mrs. Jackson checks in with Maya

Maya's dad helped her finish setting up the computer. It was 4 p.m., time for Mrs. Jackson, Maya's teacher, to call. Maya was so antsy she insisted her dad set up the computer ten minutes ahead of time.

She had combed her hair and put on her favorite denim sweatshirt, along with her bangles with baby unicorns on them.

She was signed in, waiting for the video chat to start. Suddenly, a broad grin brightened up her computer screen.

"Mrs. Jackson!" Maya yelled.

"Hello there, Maya. And how has your day been so far?"

"Just great, Mrs. Jackson. I mean, I miss school sooooo much. I miss the lunch lady, my lessons with the class, and you!"

"I miss you too, Maya, and all of my students. Did you get a chance to get outside for some fresh air?"

"Oh yes, we got out for a family walk, me and Mom played ladder ball in the yard, and Harlan kept me pretty busy."

Mrs. Jackson laughed. "I'm sure he did. That is one happy dog."

Just then, Harlan jumped, placed his front paws on the computer table and stuck his face close to the monitor.

"Harlan! Get down!" Maya yelled. "Mom, Harlan is in the way!"

Mom came running. She shooed Harlan away and got in front of the monitor herself.

"How are you today, Mrs. Jackson? Thanks so much for checking in on Maya. She loves these chats."

"That's what I love to hear. I really hope we can get back together this school year and make up for what we've missed.

"Oh, boy," Maya laughed. "I can't wait!"

Maya's mom chuckled, said her goodbyes, and led Harlan away.

"How are you handling this time away from school, and social distancing, Maya?"

"OK," she hung her head.

"I mean really. You can talk about it if it makes you feel better."

"Mom says this too shall pass. Dad says the doctors and scientists are hard at work. My brother and I just have to do our part to flatten the curve by starving the coronavirus."

Mrs. Jackson smiled. "That's very good, Maya. That's a good understanding of what we face. Just know that this is happening all over the world. We have people who get sick."

She cleared her throat. "It's important to know that many, many people get better. We want to keep away from each other for a while longer, so we can all get back to school and work in a healthy way."

"Yes, ma'am, Mrs. Jackson. I'm washing my hands an extra-long time and helping Mom and Dad dis-in-far…"

"Disinfect?"

"That's the word," Maya said. "Can I ask you something? Have any of my classmates gotten sick? I worry about them."

"No, Maya. No need to worry. Everyone is healthy and doing their best. Make sure you eat well, get lots of fresh air, and take all the safety measures your mom and dad tell you to take. You'll be fine."

"Mrs. Jackson, there is one thing. I was a little sad earlier. My birthday is coming up."

"Oh, yes! I see that on my calendar."

"But, I can't have a big party like usual. It's OK. Mom says we just need to be creative."

"Then, creative we'll be. Now, let's take a few moments to review your reading and writing lesson just to make sure you're not having any troubles. And then I want you to tell me where you found those beautiful bangles!"

Maya touched her unicorn bangles and lightly shook them on her wrist.

The soft clang reassured her.

MAYA WORRIES

Later that night, Maya heard her parents speaking in hushed tones.

Her mom had tucked her in a half hour earlier. She didn't know Maya had turned her bedside lamp back on to read a few pages of her favorite book. Instead, Maya tossed and turned in bed.

She could only hear bits of the conversation between her parents.

"...Flatten the curve..."

"...Bryan saw a news report on his computer..."

"...Pre-existing conditions..."

"...State protests against lockdown..."

"I know the kids are trying to figure it out. Same as us. They're smart kids. We just have to be there for them."

"..Birthday..."

"...We just have to be creative..."

Maya fell asleep to those words.

Our Bodies Stay Home, Our Imaginations Run Free

She woke up with an idea. Her friend, Shannon lived just a few doors down. It was time for them to set up a "six-feet-away play date."

Shannon was one year older than Maya and would help her figure out what to do for her birthday. Of course, Shannon would be invited, so she would be especially excited to come up with ideas.

* * * *

The next day after school lessons were finished, Shannon's mom came over to Maya's house with her daughter. They had arranged a time when Maya's mom could take a break.

It was lunchtime. The two moms sat on the front porch swing and chatted with their masks on.

Maya's mom had decided to wear a homemade cotton pleated mask her friend had sewn. The bright red, pink and blue pattern made her look festive.

Shannon's mom wore a floral pattern mask with navy blue, silver and gold tones. She looked like a church lady who had found her hat too small, and plopped it on her face instead.

Maya wore her favorite: a cotton pleated mask with a tiny unicorn horn sewn on the right side. Shannon's mask was rainbow colored. They were getting used to talking loud enough to hear one another through their masks.

Maya sat on the tiny steps leading up to her front walk, which were just below the steps leading to the front porch. Her lunch sat next to her: a turkey sandwich, chips, and a cherry juice box.

Shannon sat six feet away, legs dangling from her large plastic pull wagon. Her mom had brought her lunch over. The girls munched happily, with a small bottle of hand sanitizer placed next to each of them.

"What do you want to do for your birthday?" Shannon asked.

"That's why you're here. What do you think would work with coronavirus all around?"

"Well, we can't do anything that would help the virus. So, no big group of kids, no hugging and kissing…"

"Eww!" yelled Maya.

"Yeah, we wouldn't kiss anyway. For sure, not boys! Also, no hugging," Shannon said.

"Maybe games in the yard?"

"What kind of games could we play and still stay six feet away?"

"Hmmm. Let me think," Maya said.

They both turned their heads at the sound of a jingling dog tag. Walking in their direction was a fluffy, white bichon. The owner was a tall redhead. She wore a purple and white polka dot shirt, purple shorts, and a matching polka dot mask.

Our Bodies Stay Home, Our Imaginations Run Free

"Your mask is awesome," Maya shouted. "Who would have thought of polka dots? It matches your outfit! Purple is my favorite color!" She turned her head and shouted, "Mom, can I have a purple and white polka dot face mask?"

Maya's mom looked up with a mouth full of sandwich and nodded briefly. She noted the stranger, checked for a mask, and continued her conversation with Shannon's mom.

The lady in the purple polka dotted mask and outfit smiled and continued past. Her dog sniffed the air and trotted along.

The kids kept chatting. Walking toward them was a neighbor from down the street, strolling along with his chihuahua. The man looked tired in his baggy red sweatpants and an old faded gray sweatshirt.

"Hey," Shannon said. "Your mask covers almost your whole face. But your green eyes are very pretty. They match your green Crocs."

The man stopped for a moment, blinked in surprise, then smiled and continued on his way.

"We can figure out the party, while we check out the face mask fashion parade," Maya giggled.

Shannon sipped her juice. "My dad says just make sure the mask covers your face and nose so those pesky particles can't get in."

"Ooh, ooh, here comes another walker." Maya pointed.

The girls watched as a walker without a dog approached. He looked like a middle-aged man attempting power walking...for the first time. With his bald head, pumping arms, and determined stride, he was kicking up quite a sweat.

"Hello, sir," Shannon began, "Your cap and your mask make you look like a new superhero. We'll think up a name and will tell you tomorrow, if you walk by again. Bring a dog, if you have one."

The man laughed, saluted, and hurried along.

"Speaking of dogs," Maya said. "I wonder if they can sniff out coronavirus?"

"Ask your Mom and Dad, or Mrs. Jackson."

"I will."

It's Maya's Birthday!

Maya woke up on the day of her eighth birthday.

She yawned and stretched. She felt different. Then, she remembered. She had gone to sleep feeling sad, even after her mom and dad had given her big hugs before sending her off to bed.

"When you wake up, you'll be a year older. Eight years old is special," her mom said.

"Stop trying to catch up to me!" Bryan had teased. "I'm always going to be your big brother."

She was finally able to fall asleep when her dad reassured Maya that like the Tooth Fairy, the birthday wizards were still hard at work. Coronaviruses couldn't stop them. She just needed to believe.

Maya was happy at the thought of seeing her grandparents with ice cream on their next video call. Her family was going to surprise them by wearing the masks they had made.

After learning that their local hospitals were running low on masks, Maya's mom had agreed they could start a family project to help out their community.

The family committed to spending one to two hours each day making the no-sew cloth masks with material left over from one of Mom's craft projects.

Harlan entered the room carrying something in his mouth. He jumped onto her bed and deposited the item on her lap.

"What have you got there, Harlan?" Maya asked. She picked up the item and examined it. "It's a crown with unicorns all around it!"

Maya jumped out of bed, threw on her robe and slippers, and raced into the bathroom to adjust her crown. She smiled widely, tilting her head back and forth.

She hurriedly brushed her teeth and washed her hands before heading downstairs.

Her mom, dad and Bryan were already in the kitchen, hard at work. The smell of blueberry pancakes, bacon, and coffee filled the air.

"Right this way, Queen," Mom said, ushering her to a seat. Floating above her makeshift throne were eight large colorful helium-filled balloons sporting all the colors of the rainbow, with her name stamped on each one in gold.

"Wow," Maya said, looking all around her.

Her dad rushed over with a large glass of orange juice, followed by Bryan bearing a stack of blueberry pancakes, bacon, and a jumbo iced cupcake. It was bright yellow, with colorful multi-colored sprinkles on top.

"Yum. Thank you," Maya said.

"Let us get our plates and we'll sing to the birthday girl."

With her family surrounding her, Maya felt a warm glow in her stomach. For the moment, she forgot all about coronavirus, surrounded by the love of her family.

"I'll start," Bryan announced. *"Happy birthday to you…"*

Everyone joined in. *"Happy birthday dear Maya, Happy birthday to you. How old are you? How old are you?"*

"I'm eight years old!" Maya yelled. "Let's eat!"

The birthday tune was replaced by lots of chatter and clanking as the family enjoyed the birthday breakfast.

"I can't wait to see Grandma and Grandpa," Maya said in between bites.

When Maya bent down to pet Harlan, her mom and dad shared a look between them.

Bryan noticed and had to cover his mouth to keep from smiling.

Minutes later, everyone grabbed their favorite cupcake flavor from the platter perched on the kitchen counter. Mom reached for a candle for Maya's cupcake and lit it.

"Say a wish on this special eighth birthday."

Maya closed her eyes, and thought deeply, before blowing out the candle.

"Yay!" Bryan yelled. "Let's eat!"

Maya pulled out the candle and took a bite of her cupcake. Before she knew it, she had eaten half of it. "That was delicious. I'll save the rest for later. Thanks, everyone, for my great birthday breakfast."

"Our pleasure. OK, Dad and I will take care of clearing the table. We want you two to get dressed and meet us back downstairs for the next special surprise," mom said.

"Another surprise?" Maya grinned.

"Do we have to?" Bryan pleaded.

With one look from Mom, Bryan and Maya headed upstairs.

* * * * * *

Minutes later, Maya came out of her bedroom with her favorite unicorn shirt, faded jeans, and glittery peach sneakers. That's when she heard it.

"Sirens?" she asked herself.

Once she got downstairs, her mom and dad walked toward the front door and flung it open. Harlan was at their heels. They beckoned for her to follow them outside. Bryan quickly joined them.

Coming down the street was a police car with its siren flashing and whooping, followed by a yellow convertible driven by...

"Mrs. Jackson?" Maya asked, jumping up and down.

Maya's mom clapped her hands, seeing her daughter's joy.

Mrs. Jackson waved heartily, thrilled to see Maya in person rather than on a computer monitor. She drove by slowly, so everyone could read the sign on her car.

STAY SAFE.
MRS. JACKSON DEMANDS IT!

Maya kept waving furiously. Passing in front of Maya and her family was a line of cars, all at least six feet apart, with two signs taped to each car.

Each sign began:

From Mrs. Jackson's second grade class, presenting (followed by a child's name).

First came Shannon!

"You knew about this!" Maya yelled at her.

"I know how to keep a secret!" Shannon yelled back, causing Maya's family to bounce with laughter.

Shannon's second sign read:

Coronavirus will not last forever!

Next up was Lily Jones.

Keep your chin up.

Lily was followed by Michael Becker.

See you soon in class. Six feet away.

Michael was followed by Johnny Davis.

Wash your hands like someone's life depends on it!

Johnny was followed by Deisha Collins.

My behavior protects you.
Your behavior protects me.

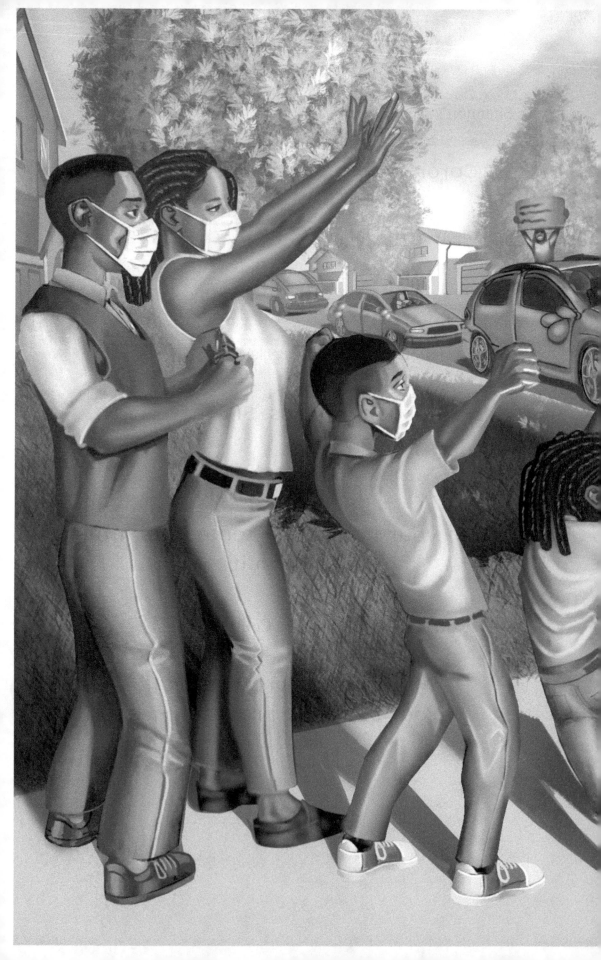

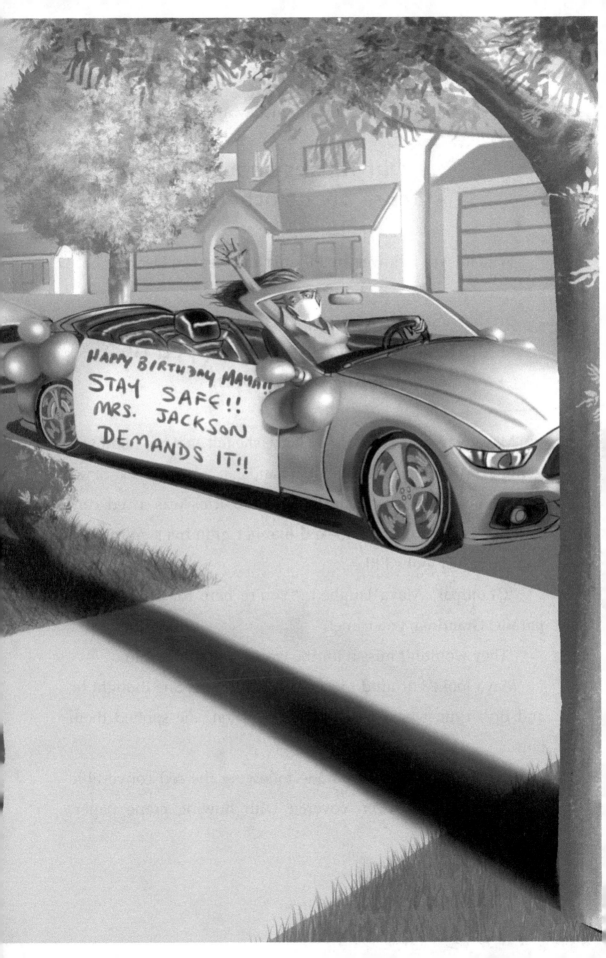

Deisha was followed by William Haward.

Our masks show we care about others.

William was followed by Monnia and Heaven Hearts.

Sending you big kisses and candy-filled wishes, wrapped up inside a unicorn.

Maya waved at everyone so hard, she felt as if her hand was going to fall off. She had to switch hands.

Following her classmates in their vehicles was a red convertible. The driver's car looked like her grandpa's sporty car, and the driver looked like...

"Grandpa!" Maya laughed. "You're here for the birthday parade! Grandma, you came!"

"They wouldn't miss it for the world," her mom said.

Maya looked around to catch her dad's eye. She thought he and Bryan must have stepped inside. Then, she spotted them both.

The gray SUV in the parade following the red convertible was unmistakable, even covered with flowing crepe paper.

Colorful balloons were taped on, sporting colors of the rainbow with Maya's name stamped in gold.

The parade came to a halt. Bryan jumped out of the family SUV, holding a microphone. He turned to his dad to cue the music.

"What's he doing?" Maya asked.

"This is going to be memorable," Mom promised.

Bryan slid on a pair of cool dark sunglasses. "I'd like to dedicate this original rap tune to my little sister on her eighth birthday. I call it *The Coronavirus, Covid-19 Song.*

Back up. Don't get all up on me.
Back up. Keep your social distance. That's what they tell us.
It's important. We all need to listen. We all need to trust.

We've got a virus. Coronavirus, Covid-19, disrupting our flow.
It's hard to stay home. We have places to go.

It's not gonna last forever. It's just for a while.
We have to give our doctors and scientists time to work.
I'm asking you to please do your part and do it with a smile.

Practice your art. Read a book. Write a song.
Using your imagination, you can stay busy all day long.

Wash your hands. Wear your mask. Stay six feet away.
If you see someone too close, use your voice, and say…
Back up! Don't get all up on me.
We all need to change our ways for a while.
Do your part and do it with a smile.

"I'm out. My name is DJ Bryan. Thank you for helping us celebrate my little sister's special birthday." With that, Bryan bowed to loud applause and ran over to Maya to give her the best big brother hug she ever had.

Maya turned and saw a neighbor wearing one of the family's handmade masks. She was filming the whole parade and performance. Maya didn't think she would ever stop smiling. To her great surprise, the lead car in the parade turned the corner, and headed back down her street. The parade began all over again.

"This is my best birthday ever!" Maya said, throwing out her arms to capture everyone in a huge virtual hug.

About the Author

Lora Hyler is a former journalist for NPR and ABC affiliate radio stations in Wisconsin. She lives in Glendale, WI and has owned a public relations and marketing firm, Hyler Communications since 2001. She writes middle-grade children's books about multi-cultural superheroes, working on the CRISPR-Cas9 gene editing technology, who share a love of spy gadgets. The first book in the series is titled *The Stupendous Adventures of Mighty Marty Hayes*. She looks forward to meeting children all over the world once the coronavirus is defeated.

www.lorahylerauthor.com

About the Illustrator

Ian Wade is an illustrator based in St. Philip, Barbados. He is working with Lora on her *Stupendous Adventures* children's book series. His talents are on display at Instagram.com/dracanimaart